颈 肩 腰
推拿保健操
中英文对照版

Traditional Chinese Tuina Exercises for Neck, Shoulder and Waist
Chinese and English Version

主编　刘明军　陈邵涛　主译　周翔宇

Editor-in-chief　Liu Mingjun, Chen Shaotao
Translator　Zhou Xiangyu

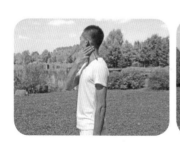
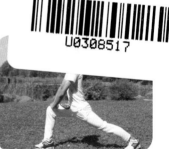

中国中医药出版社
·北京·

图书在版编目（CIP）数据

颈肩腰推拿保健操：中英文对照版 / 刘明军，陈邵涛主编 . —北京：中国中医药出版社，2017.9

ISBN 978-7-5132-4110-6

Ⅰ . ①颈… Ⅱ . ①刘… ②陈… Ⅲ . ①颈肩痛 – 按摩疗法（中医）– 汉语、英语 ②腰腿痛 – 按摩疗法（中医）– 汉语、英语 Ⅳ . ① R244.15

中国版本图书馆 CIP 数据核字（2017）第 079937 号

中 国 中 医 药 出 版 社 出 版

北京市朝阳区北三环东路 28 号易亨大厦 16 层

邮政编码 100013

传真 010 64405750

河北省武强县画业有限责任公司印刷

各地新华书店经销

*

开本 880×1230 1/32 印张 3.75 字数 89 千字

2017 年 9 月第 1 版 2017 年 9 月第 1 次印刷

书 号 ISBN 978-7-5132-4110-6

*

定价 36.00 元

网址 www.cptcm.com

前　言

随着社会的发展，学习、工作环境的改变和生活节奏的不断加快，现代人亚健康状况日趋年轻化，尤其是颈、肩、腰部的急性损伤和慢性劳损，极大地影响了人们的生活质量和工作效率。

推拿是人类最古老的医疗方法之一，经过几千年的发展，形成了其操作简便、疗效显著、无副作用、感觉舒适、易于接受等特点。由推拿按摩疗法演化而来的保健推拿，对人体疾病的预防和日常养生更是有着独特的作用。编者总结多年的针灸推拿临床、教学实践，根据推拿治疗疾病的作用原理，结合颈、肩、腰部生理特点和运动形式，传承创新、反复推敲、亲身实践、试点操作、不断改进，创编出《颈肩腰自我保健操》一书，本书出版后受到业界和读者的普遍认可和好评。应读者要求，结合目前国内外对中医保健养生的重视程度，以及我国对外交流日益丰富的现状，作者在2016年出版的《颈肩腰自我保健操》基础上编译了中英文对照版，以适应时代发展、扩大阅读人群。

本书详细介绍了颈、肩、腰各部位的推拿保健操，以及相关穴位、注意事项，通过真人动作示范，文字细解动作，使保健操生动直观、容易理解，加之动作简单、易于学习、实用性强的特点，可以作为广大读者养生保健、防治相关疾病的指导书，亦可作为从事康复、保健教学和临床工作者的参考书，实为办公、家庭必备书。

希望广大读者在使用过程中多提宝贵意见，以便再版时修订，日臻完善。

刘明军

2017年3月1日

Introduction

As our learning and working conditions evolve and our pace of life hastens with the development of the society, today we're likely to enter the sub-healthy stage at a younger age. And above all, acute injuries and chronic strains at the neck, shoulder and waist areas tremendously affect our life quality and working efficiency.

Being one of the oldest treatment approaches of mankind, Tuina has formed distinguishing features through its development for thousands of years, including its great user-friendliness, notable curative effect, zero side-effect, comfortable treatment process, and high acceptability. Derived from the therapeutic approach of Tuina, Traditional Chinese Tuina Exercises could play an important part in health promotion as well as prevention of diseases. Under the guidance of the healing mechanism of Tuina and the physiological characteristics and movement modes of neck, shoulder and waist, a Chinese version of Traditional Chinese Tuina Exercises was published in 2016 based on years of training experience and clinical practice of acupuncture, moxibustion and Tuina. Hence, there were many inheritances and innovations, deliberations and practices, as well as experiments and improvements involved in the making of the book, which earned great popularity among readers. In response to the request of the readers, the rising awareness of traditional Chinese approach of life cultivation and health preservation home and abroad, and the increased needs in today's international exchanges, we make this book bilingual based on the Chinese version, in order to keep with the trend of the time and to reach a wider audience.

This book contains guidance on how to conduct Traditional Chinese Tuina Exercises for neck, shoulder and waist, introductions to all acupoints related, as well as cautions and precautions of conduct. With the help of model demonstration and verbal elaboration, carefully selected movements in these exercises become easy to understand, follow and master. Therefore, we're confident to say that being highly accessible, practical and effective, this book could serve as a reference for educators and practitioners in the field of rehabilitation and health promotion, and as a guidebook for everyone to keep fit, prevent diseases, and treat pains. In a nutshell, it's a must-have for every office and household.

Last but not least, we sincerely welcome your comments and opinions on this book.

Liu Mingjun

March 1, 2017

目 录

Contents

I . Frequently Used Acupoints

II . Frequently Adopted Techniques

III . Traditional Chinese Tuina Exercises for Neck

IV. Traditional Chinese Tuina Exercises for Shoulder

V. Traditional Chinese Tuina Exercises for Waist

VI. Recommendations

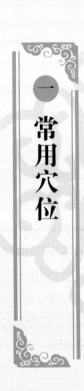

一

常用穴位

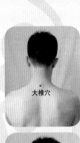

大椎穴

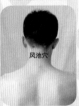

风池穴

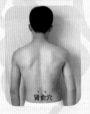

肾俞穴

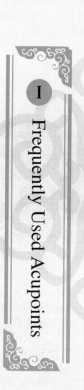

I

Frequently Used Acupoints

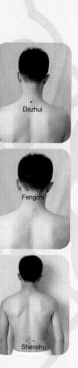

Dazhui

Fengchi

Shenshu

大椎穴

❀【定位】

在项部，后正中线上，第七颈椎棘突下凹陷中。

❀【取法】

正坐位低头时，颈后隆起最高点下方凹陷处取穴。

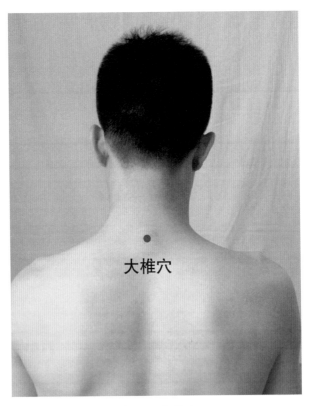

图1-1 大椎穴

GV14 (Dazhui)

❋ 【 Location 】

Acupoint GV14 (Dazhui) is located at the hollow part under the seventh crest of cervical vertebrae along the median line at the nape of the neck.

❋ 【 Positioning Method 】

Sit up, lower the head, and the acupoint could be found at the hollow part under the highest crest at the back of the neck.

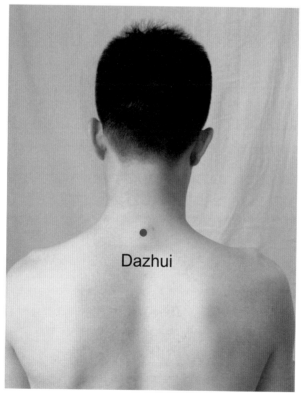

Fig 1.1　GV14 (Dazhui)

风池

【定位】

在项部，枕骨之下，胸锁乳突肌与斜方肌上端之间的凹陷中。

【取法】

俯卧位或者正坐位，项后枕骨下两侧凹陷处，当斜方肌上部与胸锁乳突肌上端之间取穴。

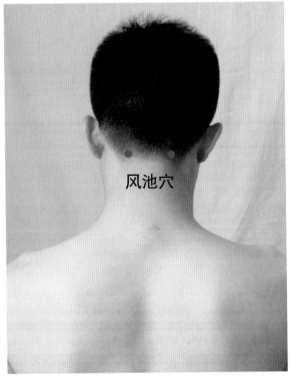

图1-2　风池穴

GB20 (Fengchi)

✤ 【 Location 】

Acupoint GB20 (Fengchi) is located at the hollow parts between the sternocleidomastoid and the upper parts of trapezius under the occipital bone at the nape of the neck.

✤ 【 Positioning Method 】

Lie prostrate or sit up, and the acupoint could be found at the hollow parts on both sides under the occipital bone between the upper ends of trapezius and the upper parts of the nutators at the back of the neck.

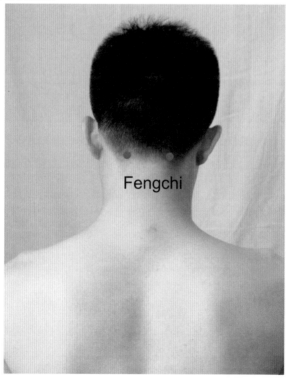

Fig 1.2   GB20 (Fengchi)

肾俞

【定位】

在腰部，当第二腰椎棘突下，旁开1.5寸。

【取法】

俯卧位，与脐相平处为第二腰椎。在第二腰椎旁1.5寸处取穴。

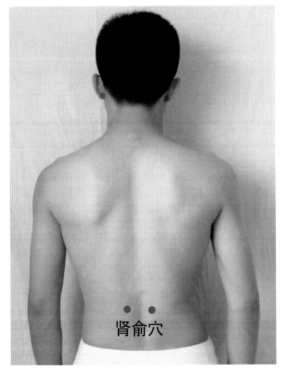

图1-3　肾俞穴

BL23 (Shenshu)

【 Location 】

Acupoint BL23 (Shenshu) is located at both sides of the second crest of lumbar vertebrae at the waist, 1.5 cun (the width of the index finger and the middle finger) away from the crest.

【 Positioning Method 】

Lie prostrate. The second crest of lumbar vertebrae on the back is opposite to the navel. Then the acupoint could be found at both the left and right sides of the crest using the index finger and the middle finger to get the right range.

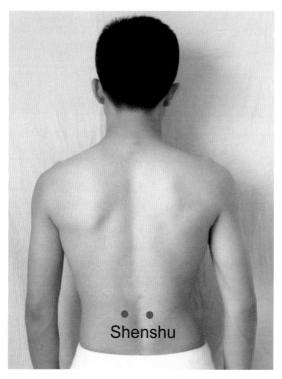

Fig 1.3   BL23 (Shenshu)

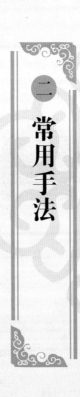

二

常用手法

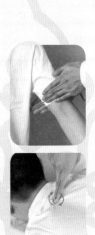

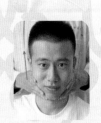

II

Frequently Adopted Techniques

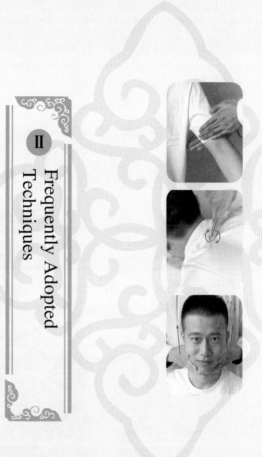

搓法

【定义】

用双手掌面夹住肢体，双手掌面着力于施术部位，做交替搓动或往返搓动，称为搓法。

【操作】

以双手掌面夹住施术部位，受术者肢体放松。以肘关节和肩关节为支点，前臂与上臂部主动施力，做相反方向的较快速搓动，并同时做上下往返移动。

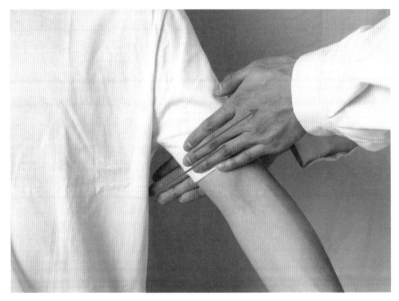

图2-1　搓法

Twisting

❀ 【 What's *twisting*? 】

Twisting is to press on the body with both palms, focusing the pressing force on the treatment area, and to massage back-and-forth or alternately.

❀ 【 How to conduct *twisting*? 】

Press on the treatment area with both hands and rapidly knead while moving upward and downward. Movements shall be driven by the forearms and upper arms, while the elbow joints and shoulder joints shall serve as the pivots. The Tuina accepter shall keep relaxed at all times.

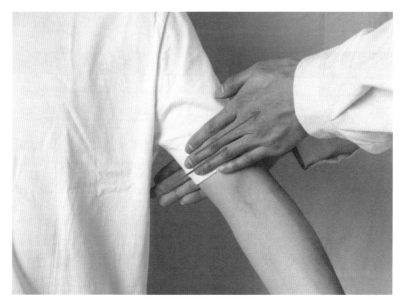

Fig. 2.1　Twisting

按揉法

※ 【定义】

　　按揉法是按法与揉法复合而成。

※ 【操作】

　　中指伸直，食指搭于中指远端指间关节背侧，腕关节微屈，用中指罗纹面着力于一定的治疗部位。以肘关节为支点，前臂做主动运动，带动腕关节和中指罗纹面在施术部位做节律性按压揉动，频率每分钟120～160次。

　　按揉法宜按揉并重，将按法和揉法有机结合，做到按中含揉，揉中寓按。

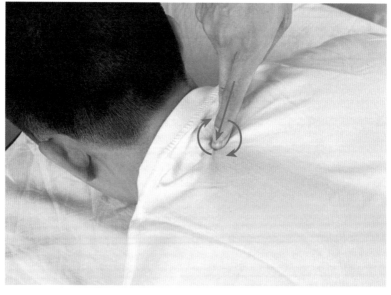

图2-2　按揉法

Pressing & Kneading

❋ 【 What's pressing & kneading? 】

This is a combination of two basic Tuina techniques as the name suggests, namely pressing and kneading.

❋ 【 How to conduct pressing & kneading? 】

Straighten the middle finger, place the index finger onto it, bend the wrist a bit, and press on the treatment area with the fingertip. Movements shall be driven by the forearm, while the elbow joint shall serve as the pivot, in order to put the wrist and the fingertip in motion to press and knead rhythmically at 120 to 160 times per minute.

Pressing and kneading share equal importance and shall be conducted as an integrated therapeutic approach.

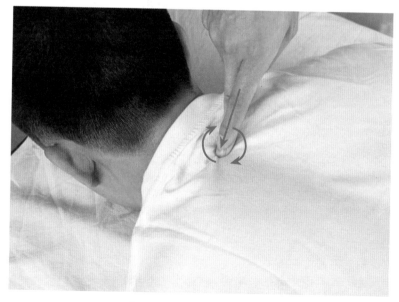

Fig. 2.2　Pressing & kneading

端提法

✤ 【定义】

　　端提法是指双手同时协同用力，向上端提头部的手法。

✤ 【操作】

　　坐位，以双手拇指端和罗纹面分别顶按住两侧枕骨下方风池穴处，两掌分置于两侧下颌部，以托挟助力。然后掌指及臂部同时协调用力，拇指上顶，双掌上托，缓慢地向上端提，使颈椎在较短时间内得到持续牵引。

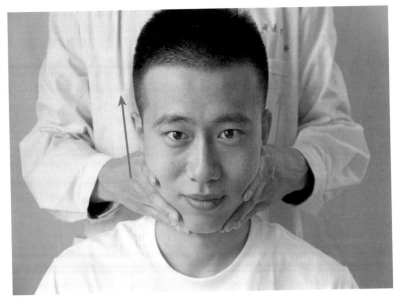

图2-3（1）　端提法（正面观）

Lifting

❋ 【 What's lifting? 】

Lifting is to put forth the force with both hands simultaneously to lift the head upward.

❋ 【 How to conduct lifting? 】

The Tuina patient shall sit up. Press acupoint GB20 (Fengchi) with fingertips of both thumbs, and hold the head by the lower jaw as a support. This should be a coordinated move of the palms, fingers and arms, of which the thumbs shall push upward and the hands shall support from under, slowly lifting in order to provide sustained traction for the cervical vertebrae during a short period of time.

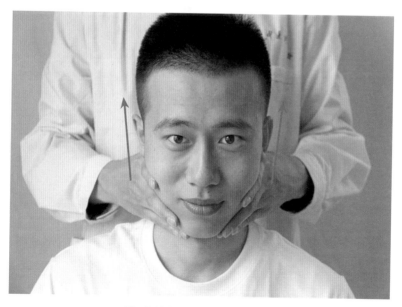

Fig. 2.3(1)　Front View of Lifting

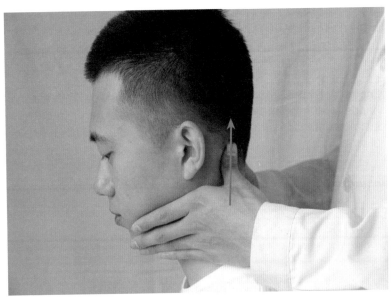

图2-3（2） 端提法（侧面观）

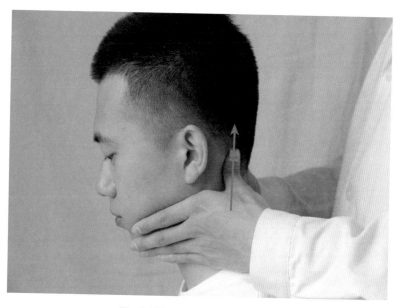

Fig. 2.3(2)   Lateral View of Lifting

抹法

【定义】

以手指罗纹面或掌面着力，紧贴于体表一定部位，做上下或左右直线或弧形曲线的往返抹动的手法，称为抹法。

【操作】

以手指或手掌面置于一定的部位上。肘关节和肩关节为双重支点，前臂主动施力，腕关节放松，做上下或左右直线的往返抹动。

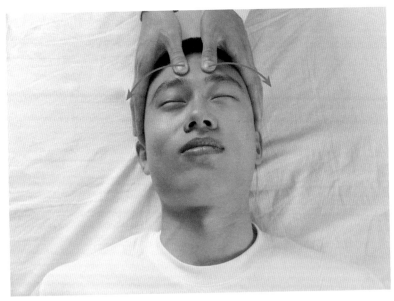

图2-4（1）　抹前额（正面观）

Wiping

❀ 【 What's wiping? 】

Wiping is to massage with fingertips or the palm back and forth horizontally, vertically or along a certain curve line.

❀ 【 How to conduct wiping? 】

Place the fingertips or the palm at the treatment area and wipe back and forth accordingly. Movements shall be driven by the forearm(s), while the elbow joint(s) and the shoulder joint(s) shall serve as the pivot.

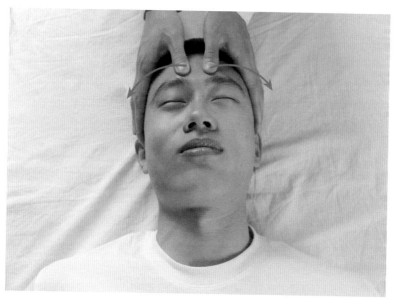

Fig. 2.4(1)　Wiping Forehead

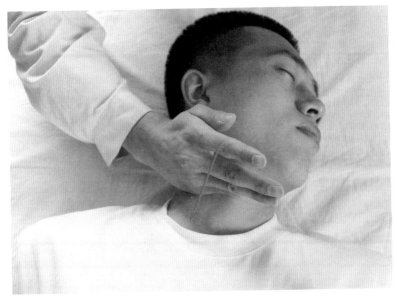

图2-4（2） 抹颈部（侧面观）

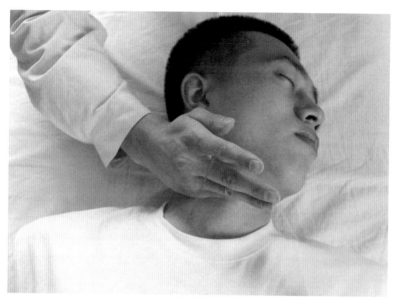

Fig. 2.4(2)   Wiping Neck

摩法

❀【定义】

　　用手掌在体表做环形摩动的手法，称为摩法。

❀【操作】

　　手掌自然伸直，腕关节略背伸，将手掌平放于体表施术部位上。以肘关节为支点，前臂主动运动，使手掌随同腕关节连同前臂做环旋或直线往返摩动。

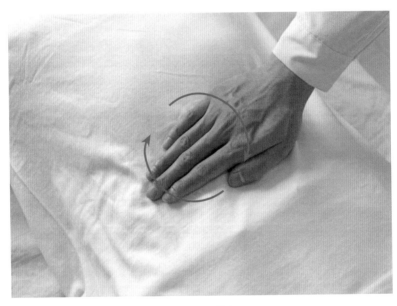

图2-5　摩法

Rubbing

🌼 【 What's rubbing? 】

Rubbing is to massage the body with the hand in circular motion.

🌼 【 How to conduct rubbing? 】

Straighten the fingers but bend the wrist a bit. Place the hand on the treatment area and rub in circular motion or back and forth. Movements shall be driven by the forearm, while the elbow joint shall serve as the pivot.

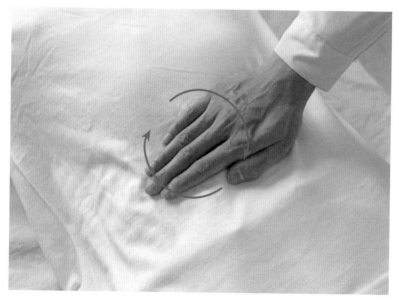

Fig. 2.5　Rubbing

点按法

❧【定义】

点按法是由点法与按法复合而成。

❧【操作】

拇指伸直，其余四指置于相应位置以助力。以拇指端着力于穴位上，前臂与拇指主动发力，进行持续性垂直向下的点按。

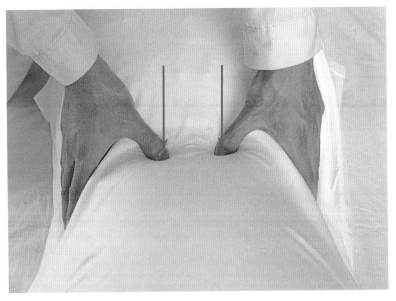

图2-6　点按法

Pointing & Pressing

✻ 【 What's pointing & pressing? 】

This is a combination of two basic Tuina techniques as the name suggests, namely pointing and pressing.

✻ 【 How to conduct point & pressing? 】

Straighten the thumbs to press vertically on the acupoints for continuous pointing and pressing, while the other fingers shall support accordingly. Movements shall be driven by the forearms and the thumbs.

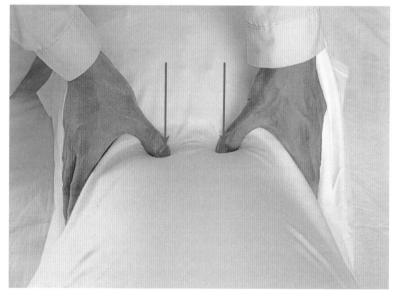

Fig. 2.6   Pointing & Pressing

叩法

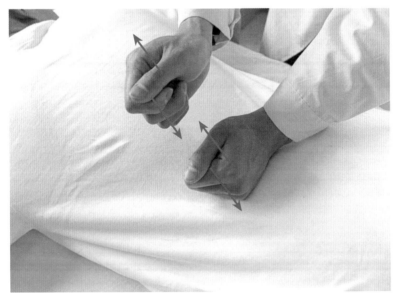

※【定义】

　　以手的尺侧，或空拳的尺侧击打体表一定部位，称为叩法。

※【操作】

　　手握空拳，腕关节略背伸。前臂部主动运动，以拳的小鱼际部和小指部节律性击打施术部位。操作熟练者，可发出"空空"的声响。

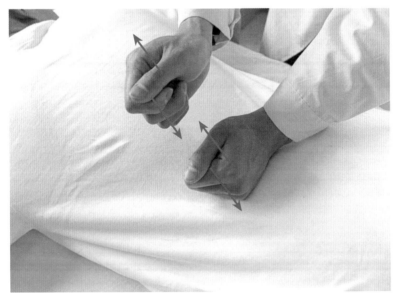

图2-7　叩法

Tapping

❀ 【 What's tapping? 】

Tapping is to knock repeatedly with the bottom of hollow fists or the thenar eminences of hands.

❀ 【 How to conduct tapping? 】

Bend the wrist a bit and rhythmically tap the treatment area with the thenars and the phalangeal joints of the little fingers. Movements shall be driven by the forearms. And there'd be pit-a-pat sound when skillful practitioners adopt this technique.

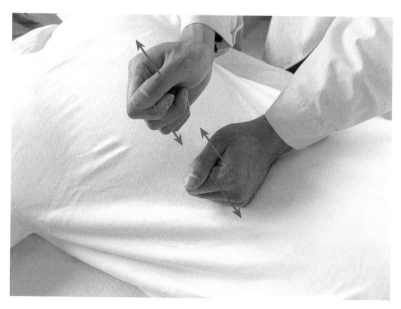

Fig. 2.7　Tapping

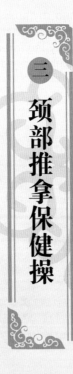

三

颈部推拿保健操

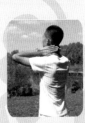

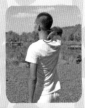

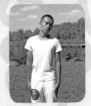

III

Traditional Chinese Tuina Exercises for Neck

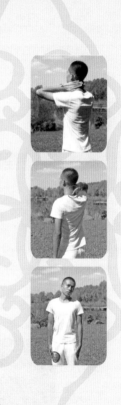

颈部操

预备动作

自然站立，双足分开，与肩等宽，双臂自然下垂，平视前方，自然呼吸，全身放松。

1. 双手搓颈

先将双手搓热，然后快速置于颈部，做前后方的推搓，以透热为度。

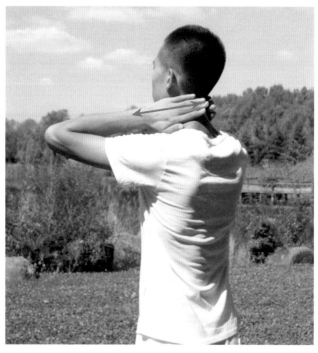

图3-1 双手搓颈

Exercises for the Neck

Get ready!

Stand still and face forward. Start with your feet shoulder-width apart and let your arms drop naturally to your side. Breathe and relax.

Step 1. Rub your neck

Rub your hands together till they get warm, then quickly hold the back of your neck with your hands and start rubbing forward and backward till it gets totally warm.

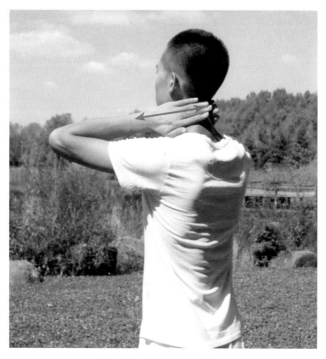

Fig. 3.1 Rub your neck

2. 按揉大椎

以一手中指置于颈后大椎穴处，按揉1分钟。

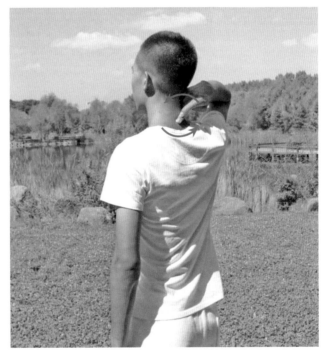

图3-2　按揉大椎

Step 2. Press & cycle on acupoint GV14 (Dazhui)

Press and cycle on acupoint GV14 (Dazhui) with the middle finger of one hand for 1 minute.

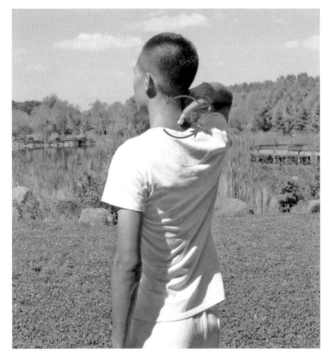

Fig. 3.2　Press & cycle on acupoint GV14 (Dazhui)

3. 左右侧颈

正视前方；先将头向左侧缓慢倾斜，至最大限度，保持5秒钟；再将头向右侧缓慢倾斜，至最大限度，保持5秒钟。左右各操作10次。

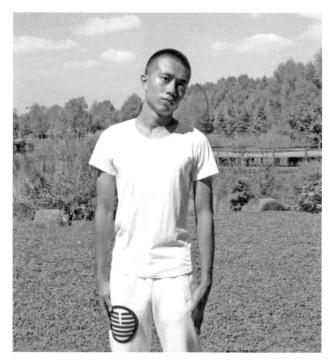

图3-3（1） 左侧颈

Step 3. Bend your head sideways

Face the front. Bend your head slowly to the left and hold it for 5 seconds, then bend your head slowly to the right and hold it for 5 seconds. Conduct 10 times to finish this step.

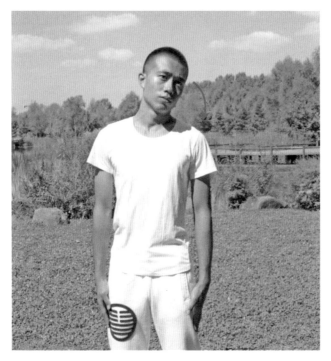

Fig. 3.3(1)　Bend your head to the left

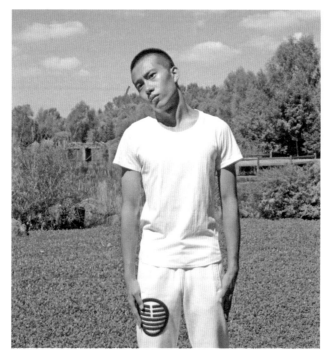

图3-3（2） 右侧颈

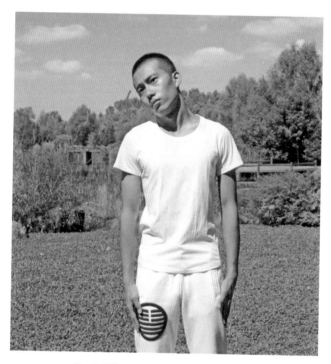

Fig. 3.3(2)　Bend your head to the right

4. 左右旋颈

目平视；分别向左、右两侧缓慢旋转头部，至最大限度后，保持5秒钟。左右各操作10次。旋转幅度可逐渐由小增大。

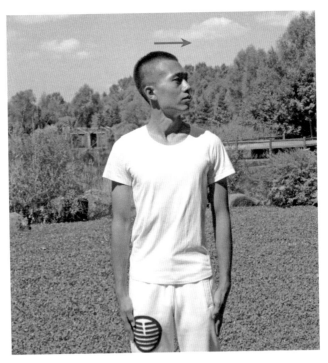

图3-4（1）　左旋颈

Step 4. Turn your head sideways

Face forward. Turn your head slowly to the left and hold it for 5 seconds, then turn your head slowly to the right and hold it for 5 seconds. Conduct 10 times to finish this step. And you may increase the extent of movement gradually.

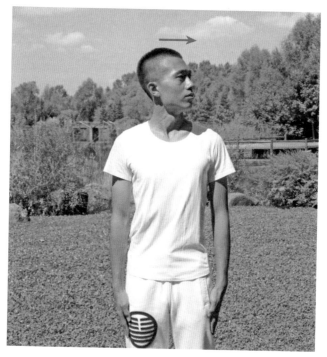

Fig. 3.4(1)　Turn your head to the left

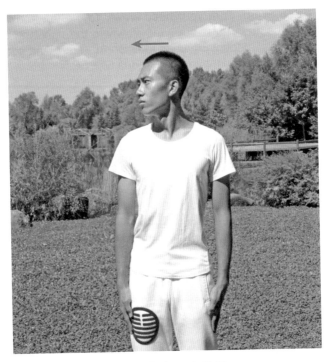

图3-4（2） 右旋颈

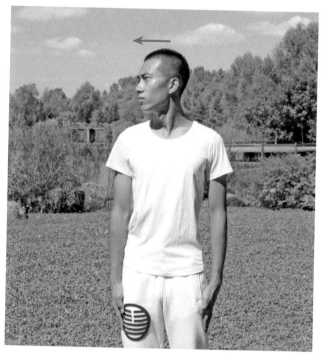

Fig. 3.4(2)　Turn your head to the right

5. 端提拔伸

　　双手拇指外展，按压两侧风池穴；余指伸直并拢，置于两侧面颊部；双手同时向上端提头部，端提至最大限度时，停留5秒钟。反复操作10次。

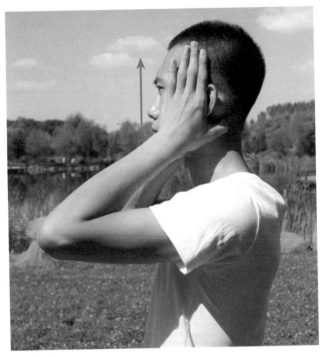

图3-5　端提拔伸

Step 5. Lift and massage the head

Press on and massage acupoint GB20 (Fengchi) with your thumbs, while straightening the other fingers to hold and lift the head from both cheeks simultaneously and hold it for 5 seconds. Conduct 10 times to finish this step.

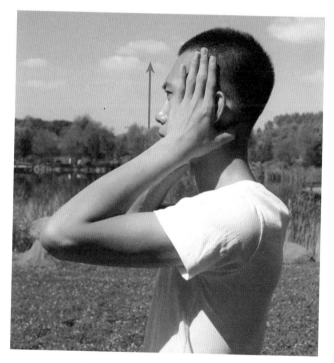

Fig. 3.5   Lift and massage the head

6. 推抹桥弓

先将头向右旋转至最大极限，眼睛看向右肩；右手食、中、无名指伸直并拢，以三指指腹自上而下推抹桥弓（耳后乳突至同侧锁骨上窝的连线）。同法操作对侧。左右各操作10次。

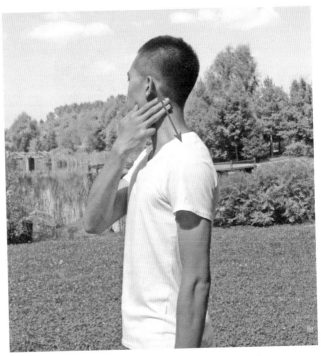

图3-6　推抹桥弓

Step 6. Wipe along the lines of Qiaogong

Turn your head to the right and look toward your right shoulder. Straighten and close the index, middle and ring fingers together to wipe along the left line of Qiaogong, which start at the root of the ear and ends at the upper concave of the clavicle, from the top-down. Turn your head to the left and wipe along the right line of Qiaogong. Conduct 10 times to finish this step.

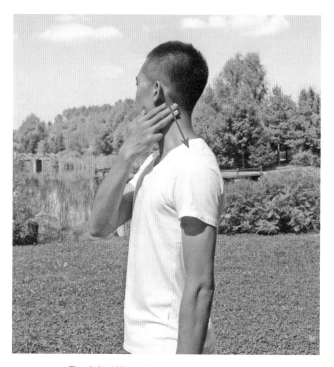

Fig. 3.6   Wipe along the lines of Qiaogong

7. 头手相争

将双手交叉置于枕部；双手向前用力，头颈向后用力，相互发力对抗8～10次，每次对抗5秒钟。

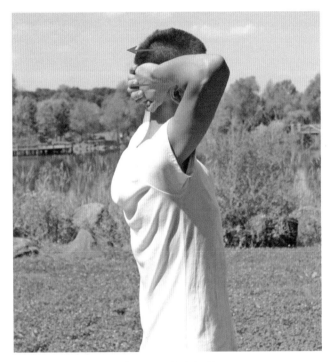

图3-7　头手相争

Step 7. Hands against the head

Put your hands behind your head and push forward for 5 seconds, while your neck pulls backward against the hands. Conduct 8 to 10 times to finish this step.

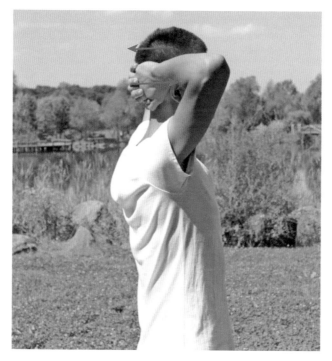

Fig. 3.7　Hands against the head

8. 仰首望天

　　目平视；将双手交叉，上举过头，掌心向上，缓慢仰视手背5～10秒；恢复起始体位，休息3～5秒钟，重复动作一次。整个动作可重复进行8～10次。

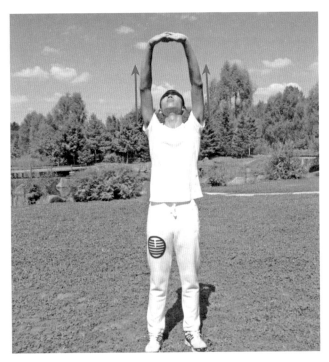

图3-8　仰首望天

Step 8. Look up at the sky

First, face forward. Raise your arms above your head with fingers interlocked and palms facing up. Look up slowly at the back of your hands for 5 to 10 seconds. Face the front again, put your arms down, and rest for 3 to 5 seconds before you start another round. Conduct 8 to 10 times to finish this step.

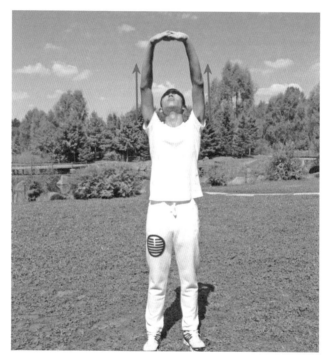

Fig. 3.8 Look up at the sky

动作要领

做上述动作时，宜持续、缓慢、均匀，切忌骤起骤停，以局部肌肉有牵张、拉紧感为宜。

功效

1. 疏经通络、行气活血，缓解颈部疼痛等不适症状。
2. 松解颈部软组织粘连，缓解相应症状。
3. 调整颈椎椎间隙，整复椎体或小关节错位。

应用

1. 预防和缓解颈椎病症状或颈部软组织慢性劳损。
2. 预防和治疗因颈部不适引起的头晕、恶心、心慌等症状。
3. 预防和治疗落枕。
4. 预防和缓解颈部肌肉劳损。

Grasping the Essentials

Pay attention to the persistency, steadiness and evenness of your movement. Avoid making any sudden moves. Mild tightness of local muscles would be appropriate.

Understanding the Mechanism

By dredging the main and collateral channels of the body and hastening the circulation of Qi and blood, symptoms such as neck pain would be relieved.

By debonding tissue adhesion at the neck, symptoms related would be relieved.

By regulating the space between intervertebral foramina, malposition of centrums as well as facet joints would be healed.

Indications

To prevent or ease symptoms of cervical spine diseases or chronicle strain of soft tissues in neck.

To prevent or treat symptoms such as dizziness, nausea and palpitation due to neck pains.

To prevent or treat stiff neck.

To prevent or ease muscle strain in neck.

四 肩部推拿保健操

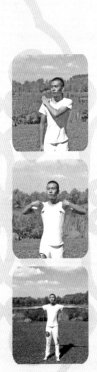

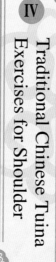

IV

Traditional Chinese Tuina Exercises for Shoulder

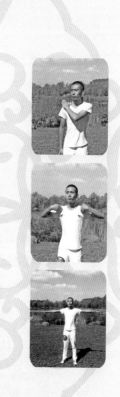

肩部操

预备动作

自然站立，双足分开，与肩等宽，双臂自然下垂，平视前方，自然呼吸，全身放松。

1. 单手摩肩

左手置于右侧肩上，轻摩肩周1～2分钟，至肩部微有热感。同法操作对侧肩部。

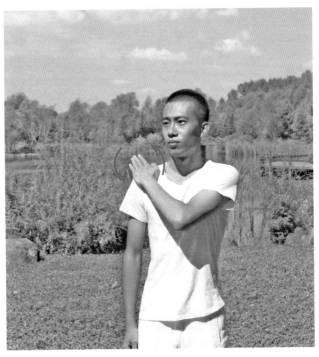

图4-1　左右旋肩

Get ready!

Stand still and face the front. Start with your feet shoulder-width apart and let your arms drop naturally to your side. Breathe and relax.

Step 1. Rub your shoulders

Gently rub your right shoulder with your left hand for 1 to 2 minutes till it gets a bit warm. Then rub your left shoulder in the same manner.

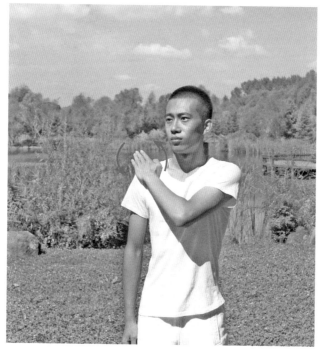

Fig. 4.1　Rub your shoulders

2. 左右旋肩

将双手置于同侧胸肩部，以肩部为轴心，分别顺、逆时针旋转上臂15～20周，旋转幅度可逐渐增大。

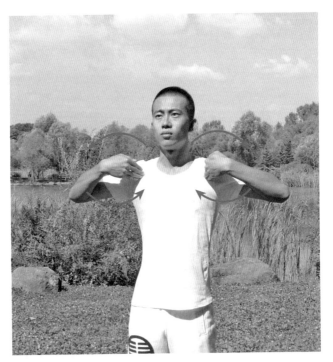

图4-2 左右旋肩

Step 2. Shoulder socket rotation

Keep your fingers on your shoulders and rotate the arms in clockwise and anti-clockwise direction for 15 to 20 times respectively. And you may increase the extent of movement gradually.

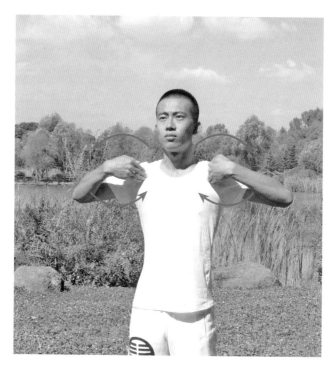

Fig. 4.2   Shoulder socket rotation

3. 外展双肩

两臂自然下垂。吸气时两手臂缓慢向上抬起、平伸，掌心向下。呼气时缓慢放下，反复操作10～15次。

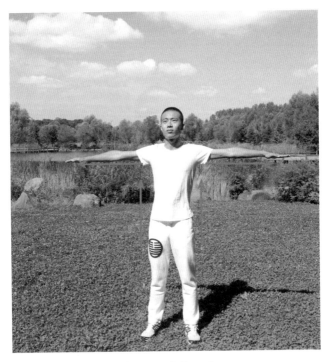

图4-3　外展双肩

Step 3. Stretch your arms sideways

Start by letting your arms drop naturally to your side. Inhale, straighten your arms and slowly raise them upwards with the palms facing down. Then exhale and put the arms down slowly. Conduct 10 to 15 times to finish this step.

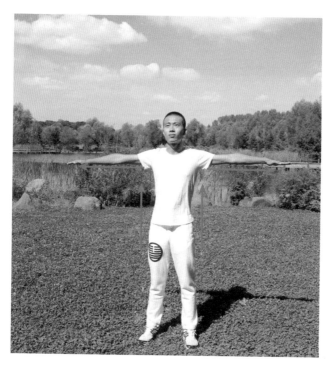

Fig. 4.3　Stretch your arms sideways

4. 托肘内牵

将右手搭于左肩上；左手托住右上肢屈曲的肘关节，并向左上方缓慢牵拉，至最大限度时停留10～15秒；反复操作8～10次。同法操作对侧肩肘部。

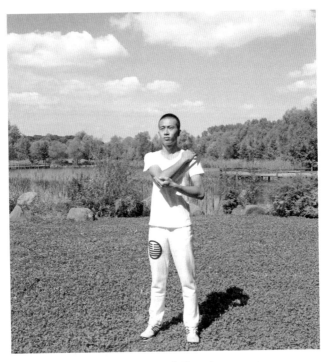

图4－4　外展双肩

Step 4. Hold your elbow and pull upwards

Start with your right hand on your left shoulder, while your left hand holds the bent right elbow & pulls slowly upwards. Hold it for 10 to 15 seconds when it reaches the limit. Then hold your left elbow and pull upwards. Conduct 8 to 10 times to finish this step.

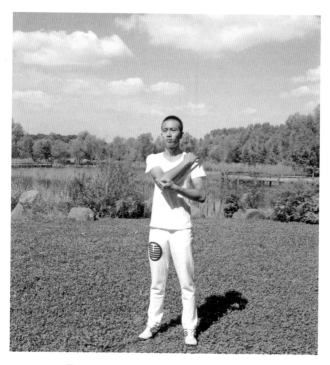

Fig. 4.4   Hold your elbow and pull upwards

5. 手指爬墙

　　面墙站立；手指做爬墙状自下而上逐步上移，直至手臂上举到最大限度。反复操作8～10次。

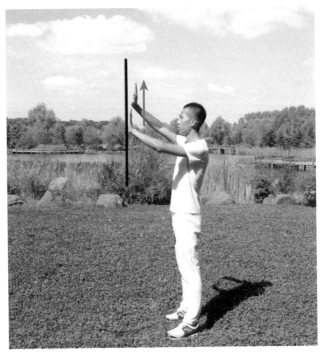

图4-5　手指爬墙

Step 5. Mock wall climbing

Stand in front of a wall. Mock the climb of the wall with your hands all the way up till your arms are straightened. Conduct 8 to 10 times to finish this step.

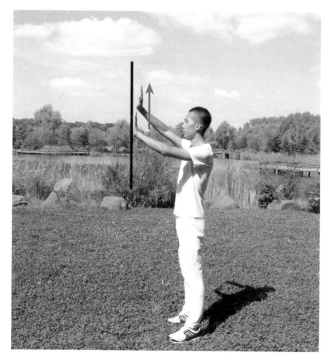

Fig. 4.5   Mock wall climbing

6. 体后拉手

　　自然站立；右臂内旋至后腰部；左手握住右手腕部，向左上方牵拉，至最大极限时停留10～15秒。反复操作8～10次。同法操作对侧。

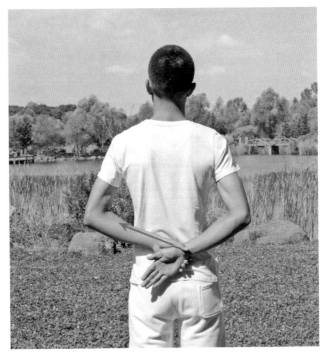

图4-6　体后拉手

Step 6. Pull your hand at the back

Start with your hands at the back as if you're in a stroll. Hold your right wrist with your left hand and pull at the upper-left direction. Hold it for 10 to 15 seconds when you reach the limit. Then pull your left hand in the same manner. Conduct 8 to 10 times to finish this step.

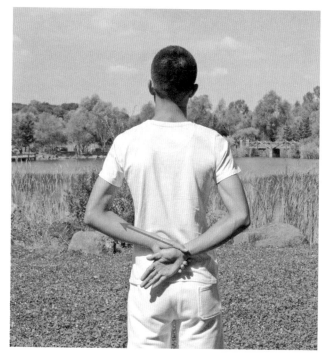

Fig. 4.6　Pull your hand at the back

7. 屈肘外旋

　　背靠墙站立；双肘屈曲成直角，双手握拳，拳心向上；以上臂为轴，前臂缓慢向两侧旋转至最大限度，停留5～8秒；再缓慢恢复至起始位。如此反复操作8～10次。

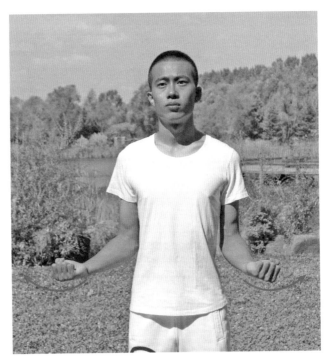

图4-7　屈肘外旋

Step 7. Bend your elbow and conduct forearm swing

Stand against a wall. Bend your elbows till your forearms are parallel to the ground. Clench your fists and swing your forearms slowly to the side. Hold it for 5 to 8 seconds when you reach the limit. Then resume your starting position. Conduct 8 to 10 times to finish this step.

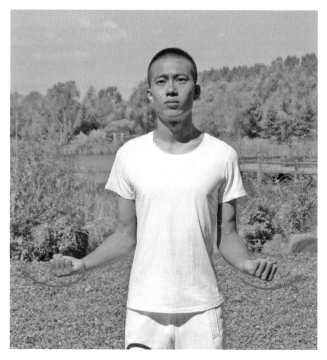

Fig. 4.7　Bend your elbow and conduct forearm swing

8. 后伸双肩

两臂自然下垂，掌心向后；吸气时双臂缓慢向后伸展至最大限度，呼气时缓慢恢复至起始位。反复操作10～15次。

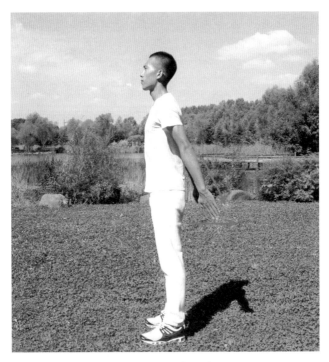

图4-8　后伸双肩

Step 8. Stretch your shoulders backwards

Start by letting your arms drop naturally to your side and your palms facing the rear. Inhale and stretch your arms backward slowly till you reach limit. Exhale and resume your starting position slowly. Conduct 10 to 15 times to finish this step.

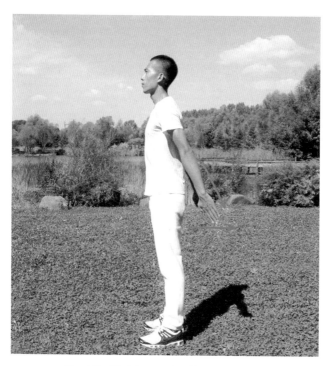

Fig. 4.8   Stretch your shoulders backwards

动作要领

做上述动作时，宜持续、缓慢、均匀，切忌骤起骤停，以局部肌肉有牵张、拉紧感为宜。

功效

1. 舒筋通络、运行气血，缓解颈肩部疼痛等不适症状。
2. 增强肌力、解除挛缩、滑利关节。
3. 缓解肩部肌肉紧张和痉挛，有利于肩关节活动。

应用

1. 各种原因所致的肩部肌肉损伤后期的康复锻炼。
2. 肩关节周围炎后期康复锻炼。
3. 颈肩综合征等引起的肩部疼痛等不适症状。

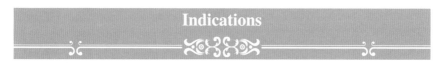

Grasping the Essentials

Pay attention to the persistency, steadiness and evenness of your movement. Avoid making any sudden moves. Mild tightness of local muscles would be appropriate.

Understanding the Mechanism

1. By dredging the main and collateral channels of the body and hastening the circulation of Qi and blood, symptoms such as shoulder pain would be relieved.

2. It strengthens the muscles, straightens the contractures and smoothes the joints.

3. By relaxing the muscles and easing the cramp, the shoulder joints would work better.

Indications

1. To be conducted as later stage recovery exercise for patients with all types of shoulder muscle injuries.

2. To be conducted as later stage recovery exercise for patients of periarthritis of shoulder.

3. To prevent or treat cervical-shoulder syndromes.

五 腰部推拿保健操

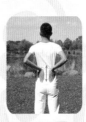

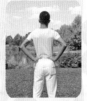

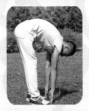

V

Traditional Chinese Tuina Exercises for Waist

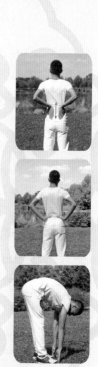

腰部操

预备动作

自然站立，双足分开，与肩等宽，双臂自然下垂，平视前方，自然呼吸，全身放松。

1. 温补肾气

双手掌置于两侧腰部，上下搓擦至局部有温热感后，停留3～5秒钟。反复操作3～5次。

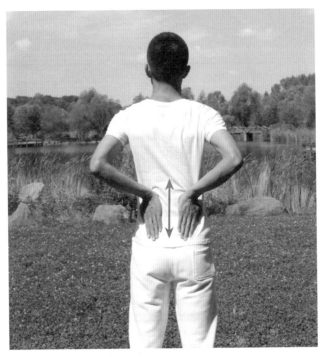

图5-1 温补肾气

Get ready!

Stand still and face forward. Start with your feet shoulder-width apart and your arms dropping naturally to your side. Breathe and relax.

Step 1. Tonify the Qi of kidney

Place your hands at both sides of your waist at the back, twist up and down till it gets warm, and then stay for 3 to 5 seconds. Conduct 3 to 5 times to finish this step.

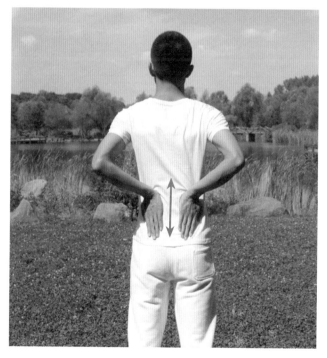

Fig. 5.1   Tonify the Qi of kidney

2. 点按肾俞

以双手拇指点按双侧肾俞穴，8～10次。

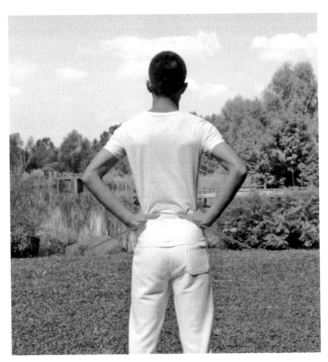

图5-2　点按肾俞

Step 2. Point & press acupoint BL23 (Shenshu)

Point and press on acupoint BL23 (Shenshu) on both sides with your thumbs for 8 to 10 times.

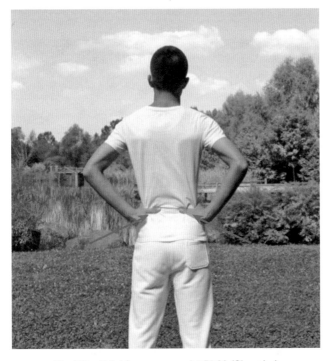

Fig. 5.2　Point & press acupoint BL23 (Shenshu)

3. 俯腰触地

双足分开与肩同宽，腰部缓慢前屈；同时双手指尖向足尖靠近，至最大限度后，停留3秒钟，再缓慢恢复至起始体位。反复操作5～8次。

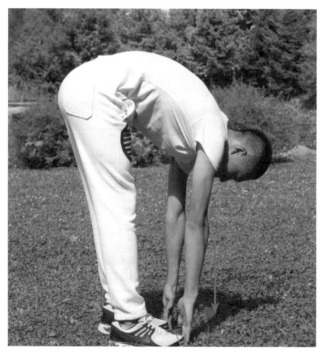

图5-3　俯腰触地

Step 3. Stand and reach

Start with your feet shoulder-width apart, bend slowly and reach for the tip of your toe. Hold it for 3 seconds upon reaching your limit. Repeat 5 to 8 times to finish this step.

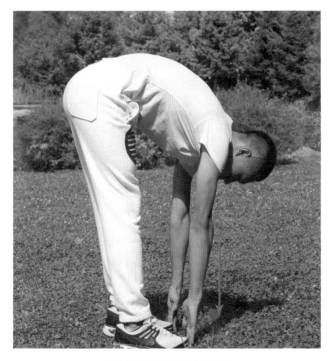

Fig. 5.3   Stand and reach

4. 腰椎后伸

双足分开与肩同宽，双手置于腰部，全身放松；腰部缓慢后伸至最大限度，保留3秒钟，再缓慢恢复至起始体位。反复操作10次。

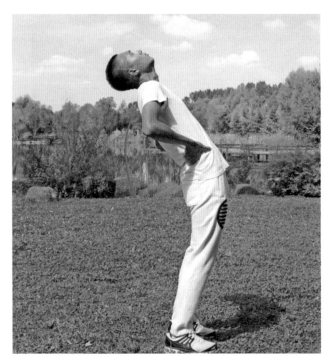

图5-4　腰椎后伸

Step 4. Stretch your lumbar vertebrae backwards

Start with your feet shoulder-width apart, your hands at your waist, and your body relaxed. Stretch your waist backward slowly till you reach the limit. Hold it for 3 seconds and resume your starting position slowly. Repeat 10 times to finish this step.

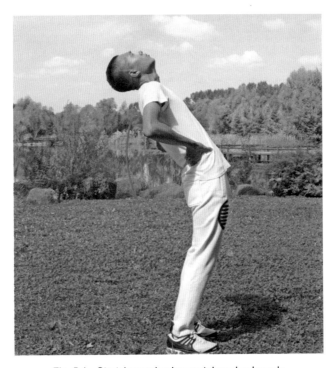

Fig. 5.4   Stretch your lumbar vertebrae backwards

5. 左右旋腰

双手叉腰，分别向左右两侧缓慢旋转腰部；然后缓慢恢复至起始位。反复操作10次。

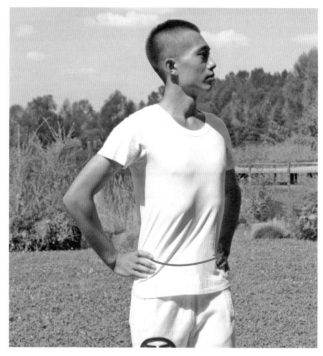

图5-5（1） 左旋腰

Step 5. Turn your waist sideways

Start with your arms akimbo, turn your waist slowly to the left. Resume the starting position and turn to the right. Repeat 10 times to finish this step.

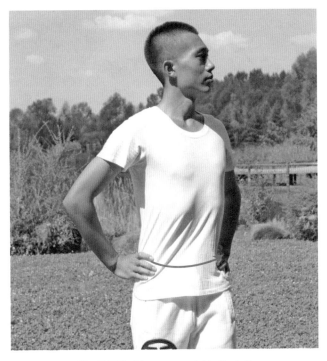

Fig. 5.5(1)　Turn your waist to the left

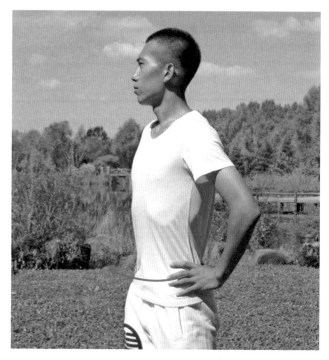

图5-5（2） 右旋腰

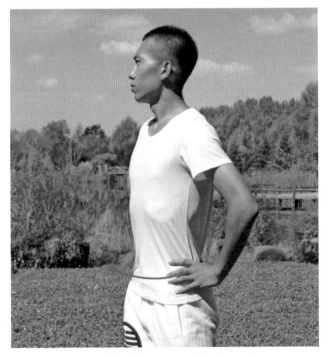

Fig. 5.5(2)   Turn your waist to the right

6. 左右屈腰

　　双手叉腰，腰部向左侧屈曲至最大限度，缓慢恢复至直立位。反复操作5～8次。同法操作对侧。

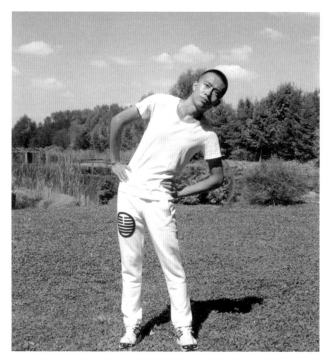

图5-6（1）　左屈腰

Step 6. Bend your waist sideways

Start with your arms akimbo, bend your waist slowly to the left till you reach the limit. Resume the starting position and turn to the right. Repeat 5 to 8 times to finish this step.

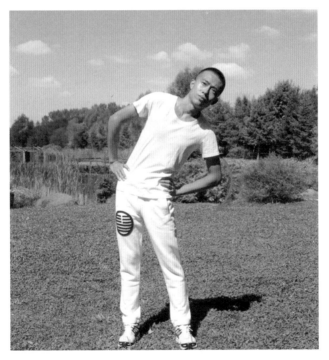

Fig. 5.6(1)　Bend your waist to the left

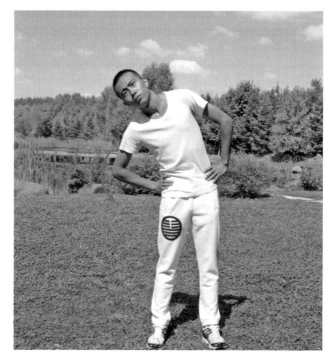

图5-6（2） 右屈腰

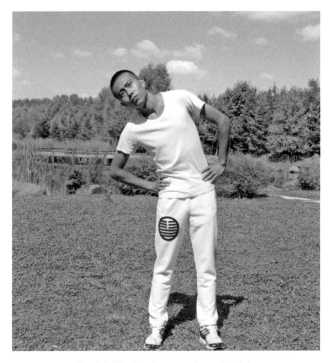

Fig. 5.6(2) Bend your waist to the right

7. 屈膝压腰

　　屈右膝，伸直左下肢，呈弓步；双手交叉置于右侧膝关节上部，下压腰部20秒；再缓慢回至原位。同法操作对侧，左右各重复10次。

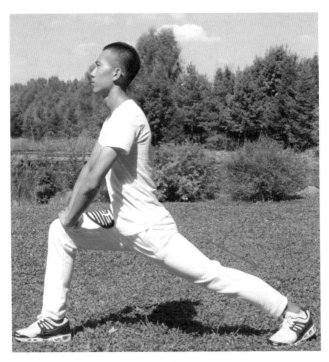

图5-7　屈膝压腰

Step 7. Bend knee and push waist downward

Start with a right lunge by bending your right knee and straightening your left leg. Put your hands on the right knee and push your waist downward for 20 seconds. Resume your starting position slowly and conduct in the same manner. Conduct 10 times to finish this step.

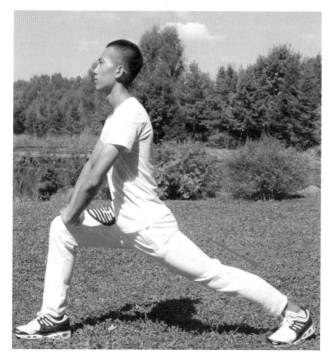

Fig. 5.7　Bend knee and push waist downward

8. 叩打腰部

双手握空拳，以虎口侧轻轻叩打两侧腰部1～2分钟。

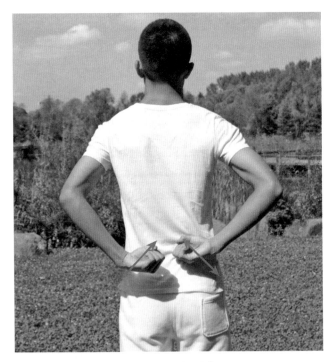

图5-8　叩打腰部

Step 8. Tap on your waist

Tap on both sides of your waist at the back with hollow fists for 1 to 2 minutes.

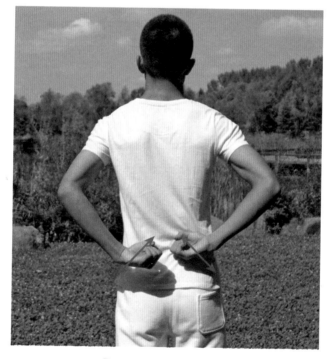

Fig. 5.8 Tap on your waist

动作要领

做上述动作时，用力宜持续、缓慢、均匀，切忌骤起骤停，以局部肌肉有牵张、拉紧感为宜。

功效

1. 疏筋通络、运行气血，缓解腰部疼痛等不适症状。
2. 缓解腰部肌肉紧张和痉挛，有利于腰椎活动。
3. 调整腰椎间隙，扩大椎间孔，整复腰椎椎体和小关节错位。

应用

1. 腰部软组织损伤后期的康复锻炼。
2. 腰椎间盘突出症后期的康复锻炼。

Grasping the Essentials

Pay attention to the persistency, steadiness and evenness of your movement. Avoid making any sudden moves. Mild tightness of local muscles would be appropriate.

Understanding the Mechanism

1. By dredging the main and collateral channels of the body and hastening the circulation of Qi and blood, symptoms such as waist pain would be relieved.

2. By relaxing the muscles and easing the cramp at your waist, the lumbar vertebrae would work more smoothly.

3. By enlarging and regulating the space between intervertebral foramina of the lumbar vertebrae, malposition of centrums as well as facet joints would be healed.

Indications

1. To be conducted as later stage recovery exercise for patients of lumbar soft tissue injuries.

2. To be conducted as later stage recovery exercise for patients of lumbar disc herniation.

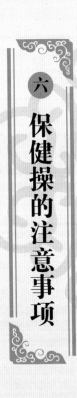

六

保健操的注意事项

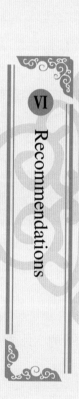

VI

Recommendations

颈、肩、腰部保健方法有多种，各有所长。本套推拿保健操是基于中医阴阳之理、经络学说和呼吸吐纳等理论，结合现代体育锻炼方法，综合传统养生武术招式简化创编而成，以期达到防病、治病、健身的目的。

　　保健操的动作要严格按照规范进行，否则不但不能起到预防、保健的作用，相反还会导致一些负损伤。所以在进行颈、肩、腰部推拿保健操时一定要注意以下方面：

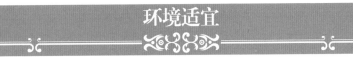

環境適宜

　　环境的适宜与否，直接影响乃至决定着功态的优劣和功效的高低。本套保健操是依据中医养生理论创编，讲究以心行气、以气运身，要求神意高度集中，以达松静空灵状态。适宜的练功环境十分重要，最好在阳光充足、空气清新、地面平坦、环境幽静的室外或室内进行。

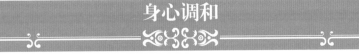

身心调和

　　调整身型：做操时，保持头面端正、身形和动作协

It's not difficult to find multiple ways based on different doctrines to promote the health conditions of the neck, shoulder and waist. The Traditional Chinese Tuina Exercises for neck, shoulder and waist introduced in this book integrates modern training exercises, the theories of Ying and Yang as well as of the main and collateral channels of human body in Traditional Chinese Medicine, the doctrines of expiration and inspiration as well as the movement of Qi, and simplified martial arts, in order to achieve our goal of health promotion and prevention and treatment of diseases.

All exercise movements should be conducted in accordance with the guidance in this book; otherwise it won't serve the purpose of disease prevention or health promotion, but cause injury. Therefore, we should pay attention to the following factors when doing the Traditional Chinese Tuina Exercises for neck, shoulder and waist.

Finding A Favorable Place for Exercising

Location is essential to the effectiveness of the exercises. Since the exercises introduced in this book is composed based on theories of traditional Chinese health promotion, it requires synchronization of the mind and the body, so as to guide the Qi with your mind and move your body with the Qi, in order to attain ease, peace, simplicity and spirituality. Therefore, it's important to pick a favorable place for exercising. An ideal site could be either indoor or outdoor, with sufficient sunshine, fresh air, flat ground and quiet surroundings.

Seeking Harmony between Body and Mind

Pay constant attention to your posture. Keep your head upright and integrate your movements to the posture. Stay

调、舒适自然，以促进人体气血正常运行，有利于精神的安静和真气的生长。全身各部放松，便于动作的施展。如果身姿不正，不仅会影响动作的规范，还会影响锻炼效果。

配合呼吸：做操时呼吸应徐徐调匀，一呼一吸自然衔接，不要刻意屏住呼吸或拉长呼吸；要腹式呼吸与胸腔呼吸相结合，最终使呼吸达到深、细、匀、长的自然状态。

意气守神：排除杂念，保持心静，专注做操，全心引导动作，心手结合。练习时适当控制速度，待动作娴熟后，逐渐在松静和缓中，体会动作过程内在的神韵，做到以意导劲，劲发随心。

规范动作

①中正安舒，柔和缓慢：即身体保持舒松自然，不偏不倚。动作尽量均匀和缓，切忌突然发力，以免造成软组织拉伤。

②连贯协调，虚实分明：即动作要连绵不断，衔接和顺，处处分清虚实，重心保持稳定。

③轻灵沉着，刚柔相济：即每一动作都要灵活自如，不浮不僵，外柔内刚，发力要完整，富有弹性。

④动中求静，动静结合：即做操时虽身体运动但内心安静，思想要集中于肢体动作。

relaxed, in order to facilitate proper circulation of blood and Qi, which could promote spiritual tranquility and generate genuine Qi for increased agility and free movements. Wrong posture could not only affect your movements, but also the effectiveness.

Regulate the rhythm of your breath. Gradually adjust your breath to a natural and regular pattern. Do not hold your breath deliberately. Adopt abdominal or thoracic breathing according to the actual need, in order to achieve a deep, gentle, steady, long and natural state of breathing.

Stay focused. Get rid of all distracting thoughts, keep calm, and focus on your movements. In tegrate your mind and your hands, so as to make every move with all your heart. Regulate the pace of exercise properly to attain a cozy, peaceful and gentle state. After learning the movements, try to feel what's behind them, to guide the energy within with your mind, and to maneuver your spiritual power rather than brute force.

Conduct the movements in accordance with the following principles:

①Put yourself at ease, but avoid leaning to either side. Keep your movements slow and steady. Avoid any sudden moves for prevention of soft tissue injury.

②Pay attention to the sequence and conduct all movements one after another like the flow of water. Regulate the application of force and keep yourself balanced.

③Do not move perfunctorily or rigidly, but dexterously, like an iron fist in a velvet glove. The application of force should be steady yet flexible, but not clumsy.

④ Attain association of activity and inertia by seeking tranquility when exercising. Focus on the movements of your body.

运动适量

　　因人而异：本保健操是依据中医养生理论创编，适合全民练习，但因个体体质、年龄、机能等存在差异，练习者应根据自己的具体情况，个性化定量练习。

　　循序渐进：该保健操注重体悟，贪快贪多不利于体悟、修身。过度锻炼会导致体力不支，动作变形，甚至劳损。做操时，要掌握用力方向的度，用力大小的度，持续时间的度，保持适当的水平锻炼。

坚持锻炼

　　保健操练习是一个循序渐进的过程，需要持之以恒，不可半途而废。只有连续的认真练习，才能不断提高，最终达到强身健体的效果。

　　坚持锻炼过程中，练习者根据季节、气候等自然变化，适当调整锻炼的量，不可死板，以免损伤身体。

自我纠正

　　在练习时，应多加观摩，相互学习交流，定期自我对

Doing What Is Possible

Firstly, individualization. Although this set of exercise, based on traditional Chinese medicine theories of health preservation, is universally applicable, one should individualize his/her workout plan that suits the age, body constitution, physical agility, etc.

Secondly, follow the principle of gradual improvement. Pay attention to the philosophy behind the exercises, rather than pushing yourself blindly, because excessive exercising would lead to exhaustion and errors. Regulate the direction, exertion and duration of your force. As you get familiar with the movements and your understanding deepens, you may build up the intensity gradually, so as to keep your exercising at a proper level.

Routinizing the Exercises

Firstly, perseverance. In this process of gradual improvement, perseverance is of the essence. It is believed that through earnest exercising and continuous improvement, you shall make a difference.

Secondly, act according to circumstances. When exercising, you should pay attention to the natural elements, such as change of seasons and weather, and adjust your exercise plan accordingly. Be flexible, so as to protect yourself from injuries.

Communicating for Improvements

Be a good observer and learner. Communicate with your fellow practitioners regularly for self-improvement;

照矫正，防止动作错误影响锻炼效果。

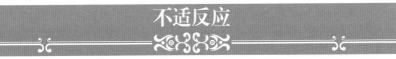

不适反应

做操时，一定要注意自身的异常变化，如果感觉不适，应该立即结束锻炼，进行适当休息，查找原因，严重者尽快去医院诊治。

otherwise effectiveness might be compromised due to errors in movements.

Dealing with Discomforts

Pay constant attention to the occurrence of anomalous change in your body. If you don't feel well, stop exercising immediately, take some proper rest, and try to find out the cause. In severe cases, visit the hospital as soon as possible, so as not to delay the treatment.